The Sou

Made Simple

Follow the Super Easy Cookbook and Guide To Learn Advanced Techniques and Wow Your Friends With Amazing Recipes.

ADAM WALSH

Furthermore, the transmission, duplication, or reproduction of any of the following work including specific information will be considered an illegal act irrespective of if it is done electronically or in print. This extends to creating a secondary or tertiary copy of the work or a recorded copy and is only allowed with the express written consent from the Publisher. All additional right reserved.

The information in the following pages is broadly considered a truthful and accurate account of facts and as such, any inattention, use, or misuse of the information in question by the reader will render any resulting actions solely under their purview. There are no scenarios in which the publisher or the original author of this work can be in any fashion deemed liable for any hardship or damages that may befall them after undertaking information described herein.

Additionally, the information in the following pages is intended only for informational purposes and should thus be thought of as universal. As befitting its nature, it is presented without assurance regarding its prolonged validity or interim quality. Trademarks that are mentioned are done without written consent and can in no way be considered an endorsement from the trademark holder.

Table of Contents

Breakfast Recipes

Sweet Potato Mix

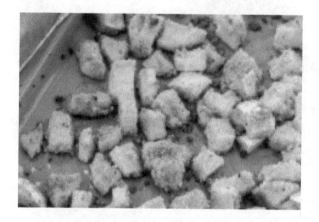

Preparation time: 10 minutes

Cooking time: 30 minutes

Servings: 4

Ingredients:

A pinch of salt and black pepper

3 tablespoons Greek yogurt

1 teaspoon oregano, dried

1 tablespoon chives, chopped

½ pound sweet potatoes, peeled, and cubed

4 eggs, whisked

½ teaspoon sweet paprika

Directions:

In a bowl, mix the sweet potatoes with the eggs and the other ingredients, whisk and pour everything into a Ziplock bag.

Seal the bag, submerge in the water oven and cook at 165 degrees F for 30 minutes.

Divide the mix into bowls and serve.

Nutrition: calories 438 fat 13 fiber 9 carbs 64 protein 26

Walnut and Berries Bowls

Preparation time: 10 minutes

Cooking time: 30 minutes

Servings: 4

Ingredients:

- 1 cup coconut cream

- 1 tablespoon raisins

- ½ teaspoon vanilla extract

- 1 cup walnuts, chopped

- ½ cup old fashioned oats

- 1 cup blackberries

Directions:

In a sous vide bag, mix the walnuts with the berries and the other ingredients, toss, seal the bag and cook in the water oven at 160 degrees F for 30 minutes.

Divide into bowls and serve.

Nutrition: calories 224 fat 12 fiber 5 carbs 15 protein 5

Chives Avocado Quinoa

Preparation time: 10 minutes

Cooking time: 30 minutes

Servings: 4

Ingredients:

 ½ teaspoon coriander, ground

 ½ teaspoon chili powder

 A pinch of salt and black pepper

 1 teaspoon chili powder

 ½ teaspoon sweet paprika

 1 cup quinoa

 2 cups veggie stock

 1 avocado, peeled, pitted and cubed

 1 tablespoon chives, chopped

Directions:

In a Ziplock bag, mix the quinoa with the stock and the other ingredients, toss, seal the bag, submerge in the water oven and cook at 165 degrees F for 30 minutes.

Divide into bowls and serve for breakfast.

Nutrition: calories 300 fat 12 fiber 6 carbs 16 protein 6

Tomato Salad and Balsamic Avocado

Preparation time: 10 minutes

Cooking time: 15 minutes

Servings: 4

Ingredients:

1 avocado, peeled, pitted and cubed

2 cucumbers, cubed

1 tablespoon balsamic vinegar

A pinch of salt and black pepper

1 tablespoon chives, chopped

½ pound cherry tomatoes, halved

1 tablespoon avocado oil

½ teaspoon rosemary, dried

½ teaspoon chili powder

Directions:

In a sous vide bag, mix the tomatoes with the avocado oil, avocado and the other ingredients, toss, seal the bag and cook at 165 degrees F for 15 minutes.

Divide into bowls and serve for breakfast.

Nutrition: calories 424 fat 23 fiber 12 carbs 42 protein 15

Apple Salad

Preparation time: 5 minutes

Cooking time: 20 minutes

Servings: 2

Ingredients:

1 teaspoon cinnamon powder

2 teaspoons raw honey

1 teaspoon vanilla extract

½ pound apples, cored and cut into wedges

¼ cup almond milk

Directions:

In a sous vide bag, mix the apples with the milk and the other ingredients, toss, seal the bag, submerge in the water oven and cook at 165 degrees F for 20 minutes.

Divide the salad into bowls and serve for breakfast.

Nutrition: calories 305 fat 19 fiber 5 carbs 29 protein 8

Pesto Zucchini Ramekins

Preparation time: 10 minutes

Cooking time: 30 minutes

Servings: 4

Ingredients:

2 garlic cloves, minced

8 eggs, whisked

½ teaspoon oregano, dried

½ teaspoon chili powder

A pinch of salt and black pepper

1 tablespoon dill, chopped

Cooking spray

2 spring onions, chopped

2 tablespoons basil pesto

½ pound zucchinis, cubed

Directions:

In a bowl, mix the eggs with the zucchinis and the other ingredients except the cooking spray and whisk well.

Grease 4 ramekins with the cooking spray, divide the zucchini mix, put the ramekins in the water oven and cook at 170 degrees F for 30 minutes.

Serve the mix for breakfast.

Nutrition: calories 356 fat 29 fiber 2 carbs 3 protein 18

Chickpeas Breakfast Spread

Preparation time: 10 minutes

Cooking time: 20 minutes

Servings: 4

Ingredients:

- 1 tablespoon lemon juice

- 1 tablespoon lemon zest, grated

- 1 tablespoon tahini paste

- ¼ teaspoon sweet paprika

- A pinch of salt and black pepper

- 1 tablespoon chives, chopped

- 2 cups canned chickpeas, drained and rinsed

- 1 cup heavy cream

- 2 spring onions, chopped

- 1 tablespoon avocado oil

Directions:

In a sous vide bag, mix the chickpeas with the cream, spring onions and the other ingredients except the oil and the tahini paste, seal the bag, submerge in the water oven and cook at 165 degrees F for 20 minutes.

Transfer the mix to a blender, add the remaining ingredients, pulse well, divide into bowls and serve for breakfast.

Nutrition: calories 203 fat 12 fiber 4 carbs 15 protein 4

LUNCH RECIPES

Pork & Zucchini Ribbons

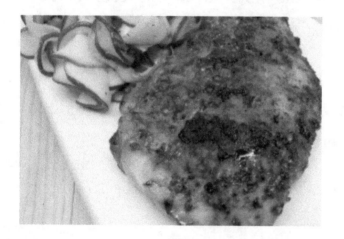

Preparation Time: 20 minutes

Cooking Time: 3 hours

Servings: 2

Ingredients:

   2 (6-ounce bone-in pork loin chops

   Salt and black pepper as needed

   3 tablespoons extra-virgin olive oil

   1 tablespoon freshly squeezed lemon juice

2 teaspoons red wine vinegar

2 teaspoons honey

2 tablespoons rice bran oil

2 medium zucchini, sliced into ribbons

2 tablespoons pine nuts, toasted up

Directions:

Prepare the Sous Vide water bath using your immersion circulator and raise the temperature to 140-degrees Fahrenheit.

Take the pork chops and season it with salt and pepper, transfer to a heavy duty zip bag and add 1 tablespoon of oil .

Seal using the immersion method and cook for 3 hours.

Prepare the dressing by whisking lemon juice, honey, vinegar, 2 tablespoons of olive oil and season with salt and pepper.

Once cooked, remove the bag from the water bath and discard the liquid.

Heat up rice bran oil in a large skillet over high heat and add the pork chops, sear until browned (1 minute per side

Once done, transfer it to a cutting board and allow to rest for 5 minutes.

Take a medium bowl and add the zucchini ribbons with
   dressing

Thinly slice the pork chops and discard the bone.

Place the pork on top of the zucchini.

Top with pine nuts and serve!

Nutrition: Calories 334, Fat 33, Fiber 3, Carbs 14,
Protein 7

Herbed Pork Loin

Preparation Time: 20 minutes

Cooking Time: 2 hours

Servings: 4

Ingredients:

1 (1 lb. pork tenderloin, trimmed

Salt and fresh ground pepper as needed

1 tablespoon chopped fresh basil + additional for servings

1 tablespoon chopped fresh parsley + additional for servings

1 tablespoon chopped fresh rosemary + additional for servings

2 tablespoons unsalted butter

Directions:

Prepare the Sous Vide water bath using your immersion circulator and raise the temperature to 134-degrees Fahrenheit. Season the tenderloin with pepper and salt

Rub herbs (a mixture of basil, parsley and rosemary all over the tenderloin and transfer to a resalable zip bag

Add 1 tablespoon of butter

Seal using the immersion method. Submerge underwater and cook for 2 hours

Once cooked, remove the bag and remove the pork from the bag

Place a large-sized skillet over medium–high heat

Add the remaining butter and herb mixture and allow the butter to heat up

Add the pork and sear it well for 1-2 minutes each side, making sure to keep scooping the butter over the pork

Remove the heat and transfer the pork to a cutting board

Allow it to rest for 5 minutes and slice into medallions

Serve with extra herbs and a sprinkle of salt

Nutrition: Calories 334, Fat 33, Fiber 3, Carbs 14, Protein 7

DINNER RECIPES

Hawaiian Pork Sliders

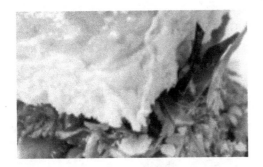

Preparation Time: 25 minutes

Cooking Time: 24 hours

Servings: 4

Ingredients:

3 tablespoons light brown sugar

3 tablespoons ground Hawaiian sea salt

2 tablespoons garlic powder

Freshly ground black pepper, to taste

3 pounds bone-in pork shoulder

1 tablespoon vegetable oil

3 tablespoons liquid smoke

1 cup pineapple juice

½ cup mayonnaise

¼ cup white wine vinegar

1 cup pineapple, diced finely

14-ounce bag coleslaw mix

2 tablespoons scallions, thinly sliced

Kosher salt, to taste

24 King's Hawaiian rolls

Directions:

Mix sugar, Hawaiian salt, garlic powder, and 2 tablespoons of black pepper together in a large bowl. Add pork shoulder and coat with sugar mixture. Cover and refrigerate for at least 12 hours.

Attach the sous vide immersion circulator to a Cambro container or pot with water using an adjustable clamp and preheat water to 150°F.

Remove pork shoulder from refrigerator and pat dry with paper towels. Discard any accumulated liquid.

In a large skillet, heat oil over medium-high heat and sear pork shoulder for 5 minutes or until golden brown on both sides. Transfer pork shoulder to a plate and set aside to cool for 10 minutes.

Place pork shoulder, liquid smoke, and pineapple juice in a cooking pouch.

Seal pouch tightly after removing the excess air. Place pouch in sous vide bath and set the cooking time for 24 hours.

Remove pouch from the sous vide bath and open carefully. Remove pork roast from pouch and place into a bowl. Set aside to cool for 20 minutes. Reserve cooking liquid in a large bowl.

With 2 forks, shred pork shoulder into bite-sized pieces. Discard any large Fat pieces and bones. Add the shredded pork to the bowl of reserved cooking liquid and toss to coat.

In another large bowl, add mayonnaise and vinegar and beat until well combined. Add pineapple, coleslaw mix, scallions, kosher salt, and black pepper and mix until well combined.

Place pulled pork and coleslaw mixture on each roll and serve.

Nutrition: Calories 471 Total Fat 32.8g Total Carb 6.1g Dietary Fiber 0.4g Protein 36g

Sweet & Spicy Pork Loin

Preparation Time: 15 minutes

Cooking Time: 6 hours

Servings: 4

Ingredients:

  2-pound pork loin roast

  1 teaspoon garlic powder

  ½ teaspoon chipotle powder

  1 teaspoon salt

  1 teaspoon freshly ground black pepper

  2 tablespoons sweet & sour duck sauce or sweet glaze of
  your choice

Directions:

Attach the sous vide immersion circulator to a Cambro
container or pot with water using an adjustable clamp
and preheat water to 153°F.

In a small bowl, mix together garlic powder, chipotle
powder, salt, and black pepper. Rub pork loin
generously with spice mixture.

Place pork loin in a cooking pouch. Seal pouch tightly after removing the excess air. Place pouch in sous vide bath and set the cooking time for 4-6 hours.

Preheat the oven broiler to high.

Remove pouch from the sous vide bath and open carefully. Remove pork loin from pouch and pat dry with paper towels.

Coat each rib section evenly with BBQ sauce and broil for 5 minutes per side.

Serve immediately.

Nutrition: Calories 471 Total Fat 32.8g Total Carb 6.1g Dietary Fiber 0.4g Protein 36g

Pork roast with milk gravy

Preparation Time: 20 minutes

Cooking Time: 6 hours

Servings: 4

Ingredients:

For Pork Roast:

¼ cup olive oil

½ teaspoon dried parsley, crushed

½ teaspoon dried oregano, crushed

Onion powder, to taste

Garlic salt, to taste

Salt and freshly ground black pepper, to taste

1½-2-pound pork sirloin roast

For Milk Gravy:

½ cup butter

⅓ cup flour

3 cups milk, either 2% or whole

Cooking liquid from pork roast

½ teaspoon beef "better than bouillon" stock (optional)

Salt and freshly ground black pepper, to taste

Directions:

Attach the sous vide immersion circulator to a Cambro container or pot with water using an adjustable clamp and preheat water to 150°F.

For pork roast: in a small bowl, mix together all ingredients for pork roast except for the roast. Rub the oil mixture generously over the pork roast.

Place pork roast in a cooking pouch. Seal pouch tightly after removing the excess air. Place pouch in sous vide bath and set the cooking time for 4-6 hours.

Remove pouch from the sous vide bath and open carefully. Remove pork roast from pouch, reserving cooking liquid into a large bowl.

For milk gravy: melt butter over medium-low heat in a medium pan. Slowly add flour, beating continuously. Cook for 2-3 minutes, continuing to beat.

While beating, slowly add milk and reserved cooking liquid. Increase heat to medium and cook until gravy becomes thick, stirring continuously. Stir in bouillon, salt, and black pepper and remove from heat.

Heat a cast iron grill pan over high heat and sear pork roast for 2-3 minutes or until completely golden brown and serve with gravy.

Nutrition: Calories 471 Total Fat 32.8g Total Carb 6.1g Dietary Fiber 0.4g Protein 36g

Ribeye with Pepper Sauce

Preparation Time: 15 minutes

Cooking Time: 7 hours

Servings: 4

Ingredients:

For Steak:

4-pounds bone-in ribeye steaks

Dry spice rub of your choice

Kosher salt, to taste

Sunflower oil, as required

For Sauce:

½ teaspoon Sichuan peppercorns

1 tablespoon butter

1 tablespoon plain flour

2 tablespoons Brandy

5 tablespoons heavy cream

Milk, as required

Salt, to taste

Directions:

Attach the sous vide immersion circulator to a Cambro container or pot with water using an adjustable clamp and preheat water to 131°F.

Season steak generously with dry rub and salt.

Place steak in a large cooking pouch. Seal pouch tightly after removing the excess air. Place pouch in sous vide bath and set the cooking time for 7 hours.

For sauce: in a pestle and mortar, crush peppercorns lightly. Heat a dry frying pan and toast crushed peppercorns until fragrant.

In the same frying pan, melt butter and stir in the flour. Add brandy and stir until a paste is formed. Add cream and stir until smooth to remove any lumps. Stir in a little milk and cook until desired thickness of sauce is reached. Stir in salt and remove from heat.

Remove pouch from the sous vide bath and open carefully. Remove steak from pouch and pat dry with paper towels.

Lightly grease a cast iron frying pan with oil and heat. Add steak and cook for 1 minute on each side.

Remove from heat and transfer onto a cutting board. Cut steak into slices, going against the grain of the meat. Serve immediately with sauce.

Nutrition: Calories 471 Total Fat 32.8g Total Carb 6.1g

Dietary Fiber 0.4g Protein 36g

Miso Glazed Beef Steak

Preparation Time: 15 minutes

Cooking Time: 18 hours

Servings: 4

Ingredients:

¼ cup brown sugar

¼ cup miso paste

¼ cup mirin

¼ cup soy sauce

2 pounds beef BBQ steaks

Salt, to taste

Directions:

In a food processor, combine brown sugar, miso paste, mirin, and soy sauce and pulse until smooth.

Transfer mirin mixture to a large bowl. Add steaks, coat with mixture, and refrigerate to marinate overnight.

Attach the sous vide immersion circulator to a Cambro container or pot with water using an adjustable clamp and preheat water to 150°F.

Place steaks with marinade in a cooking pouch. Seal pouch tightly after removing the excess air. Place pouch in sous vide bath and set the cooking time for 18 hours. Cover the sous vide bath with plastic wrap to minimize water evaporation. Add water intermittently to keep the water level up.

Remove pouch from the sous vide bath and open carefully. Remove steaks from pouch, reserving cooking liquid in a pan.

Place pan over stove and cook until the liquid reduces by half.

Preheat grill to high heat.

Season steaks with salt. Coat with reduced sauce and grill until desired doneness is reached.

Nutrition: Calories 471 Total Fat 32.8g Total Carb 6.1g Dietary Fiber 0.4g Protein 36g

Porterhouse Steak

Preparation Time: 15 minutes

Cooking Time: 1 hour

Servings: 4

Ingredients:

2 tablespoons organic butter

8 fresh thyme sprigs, divided

1 fresh rosemary sprig, split in half

2 bay leaves

2 (1-inch thick) porterhouse steaks

Kosher salt and cracker black pepper, to taste

Directions:

Attach the sous vide immersion circulator to a Cambro container or pot with water using an adjustable clamp and preheat water to 126°F.

In a small pan, melt butter over medium heat and cook herb sprigs and bay leaves for 3 minutes. Remove from heat and set aside to cool.

Season porterhouse steaks with salt and fresh cracked black pepper.

In 2 large cooking pouches, evenly divide steaks and butter mixture so each pouch contains 1 steak, 4 thyme sprigs, ½ rosemary sprig, and 1 bay leaf. Seal pouches tightly after removing the excess air. Place pouch in sous vide bath and set the cooking time for 1 hour.

Preheat grill to high heat.

Remove pouches from the sous vide bath and open carefully. Remove steaks from pouches, reserving cooking liquid in a baking tray. Pat dry steaks with paper towels.

Place steaks on the grill for 15 seconds then rotate 90 degrees and grill for another 15 seconds. Flip and repeat the process.

Remove steaks from grill and transfer to the baking tray of reserved cooking liquid. Coat steaks evenly with cooking liquid.

Serve immediately.

Nutrition: Calories 471 Total Fat 32.8g Total Carb 6.1g Dietary Fiber 0.4g Protein 36g

MEAT RECIPES

Peppery Lemon Lamb Chops With Papaya Chutney

Preparation Time: 1 hour 15 minutes

Cooking Time: 25-75 minutes

Servings: 4

Ingredients:

- 8 lamb chops
- 2 tbsp olive oil
- ½ tsp Garam Masala
- ¼ tsp lemon pepper
- Dash of garlic pepper
- Salt and black pepper to taste
- ½ cup yogurt
- ¼ cup fresh cilantro, chopped
- 2 tbsp papaya chutney
- 1 tbsp curry powder

1 tbsp onion, finely chopped

Chopped cilantro for garnish

Directions:

Prepare a water bath and place the Sous Vide in it. Set to 138 F. Brush the chops with olive oil and top with the Garam Masala, lemon pepper, garlic powder, salt and pepper. Place the chops in a vacuum-sealable bag. Release air by the water displacement method, seal and submerge the bag in the water bath. Cook for 1 hour.

Meanwhile, prepare the sauce mixing the yogurt, papaya chutney, cilantro, curry powder and onion. Transfer to a plate. Once the timer has stopped, remove the lamb and dry it.

Heat the remaining oil in a skillet over medium heat and sear the lamb for 30 seconds per side. Strain with a baking sheet. Serve the chops with the yogurt sauce. Garnish with cilantro.

Nutrition: Calories 352, Fat 5, Fiber 3, Carbs 7, Protein 5

Spicy Lamb Kebabs

Preparation Time: 2 hours 20 minutes

Cooking Time: 25-75 minutes

Servings: 4

Ingredients:

1 pound leg lamb, boneless, cubed

2 tbsp chili paste

1 tbsp olive oil

Salt to taste

1 tsp cumin

1 tsp coriander

½ tsp black pepper

Greek yogurt

Fresh mint leaves for servings

Directions:

Prepare a water bath and place the Sous Vide in it. Set to 134 F. Combine all the ingredients and place it in a vacuum-sealable bag. Release air by the water displacement method, seal and submerge the bag in the water bath. Cook for 2 hours.

Once the timer has stopped, remove the lamb and dry it. Transfer the lambs to a grill and cook for 5 minutes. Set aside and allow resting for 5 minutes. Serve with Greek yogurt and mint.

Nutrition: Calories 352, Fat 5, Fiber 3, Carbs 7, Protein 5

Herby Lamb With Veggies

Preparation Time: 48 hours 30 minutes

Cooking Time: 25-75 minutes

Servings: 8

Ingredients:

2 lamb shanks, bone-in

1 can diced tomatoes with juice

1 cup veal stock

1 cup onion, finely diced

½ cup celery, finely diced

½ cup carrot, finely diced

½ cup red wine

2 sprigs fresh rosemary

Salt and black pepper to taste

1 tsp ground coria

1 tsp ground cumin

1 teaspoon thyme

Directions:

Prepare a water bath and place the Sous Vide in it. Set
to 149 F.

Combine all the ingredients and place it in a vacuum-sealable bag. Release air by the water displacement method, seal and submerge the bag in the water bath. Cook for 48 hours.

Once the timer has stopped, remove the shanks and transfer to a plate and allow cooling for 48 hours. Clean the lamb removing the bones and the Fat then chop in bites. Transfer the no-Fat cooking juices and bites lambs to a saucepan. Cook for 10 minutes over high heat until the sauce thickens. Serve.

Nutrition: Calories 352, Fat 5, Fiber 3, Carbs 7, Protein 5

Garlic Rack Of Lamb

Preparation Time: 1 hour 30 minutes

Cooking Time: 25-75 minutes

Servings: 4

Ingredients:

2 tbsp butter

2 racks of lamb, frenched

1 tbsp olive oil

1 tbsp sesame oil

4 garlic cloves, minced

4 fresh basil sprigs, halved

Salt and black pepper to taste

Directions:

Prepare a water bath and place the Sous Vide in it. Set to 130 F. Season the rack lamb with salt and pepper. Place the rack in a large vacuum-sealable bag.

Release air by the water displacement method, seal and submerge the bag in the water bath. Cook for 1 hour and 15 minutes.

Once the timer has stopped, remove the rack and pat dry with kitchen towel. Heat the sesame oil in a skillet over high heat and sear the rack for 1 minute per side. Set aside.

Put 1 tbsp of butter in the skillet and add the half of garlic and half of basil. Top over the rack. Sear the rack for 1 minute. Turn around and pour more butter. Repeat the process for all the racks. Cut the rack in single pieces and serve 4 pieces in each plate. Season with the salt.

Nutrition: Calories 352, Fat 5, Fiber 3, Carbs 7, Protein 5

Herb Crusted Lamb Rack

Preparation Time: 3 hours 30 minutes

Cooking Time: 25-75 minutes

Servings: 6

Ingredients:

Lamb Rack:

3 large racks of lamb

Salt and black pepper to taste

1 sprig rosemary

2 tbsp olive oil

Herb Crust:

2 tbsp fresh rosemary leaves

½ cup macadamia nuts

2 tbsp Dijon mustard

½ cup fresh parsley

2 tbsp fresh thyme leaves

2 tbsp lemon zest

2 cloves garlic

2 Egg whites

Directions:

Make a water bath, place the Sous Vide in it, and set to
140 F.

Pat dry the lamb using a napkin and rub the meat with
salt and black pepper. Place a pan over medium heat
and add olive oil. Once it has heated, sear the lamb
on both sides for 2 minutes.

Remove and place aside. Add garlic and rosemary to the
pan, toast for 2 minutes and pour over the lamb.
Leave lamb to sit and cool for 5 minutes.

Place lamb, garlic, and rosemary in a vacuum-sealable
bag, release air by the water displacement method
and seal the bag. Submerge the bag in the water bath.

Set the timer to cook for 3 hours. Once the timer has
stopped, remove the bag, unseal it and take out the
lamb. Whisk the egg whites and place aside.

Blend the remaining listed herb crust ingredients using a
blender and place aside. Pat dry the lamb using a
napkin and brush the meat with the egg whites. Dip
into the herb mixture and coat graciously.

Place the lamb racks with crust side up on a baking sheet.
Bake in an oven for 15 minutes. Gently slice each
cutlet using a sharp knife. Serve with a side of pureed
vegetables.

Nutrition: Calories 352, Fat 5, Fiber 3, Carbs 7, Protein 5

Popular South African Lamb & Cherry Kebabs

Preparation Time: 8 hours 40 minutes

Cooking Time: 25-75 minutes

Servings: 6

Ingredients:

¾ cup white wine vinegar

½ cup dry red wine

2 onions, chopped

4 garlic cloves, minced

Zest of 2 lemons

6 tbsp brown sugar

2 tbsp caraway seeds, crushed

1 tbsp cherry jam

1 tbsp corn flour

1 tbsp curry powder

1 tbsp grated ginger

2 tsp salt

1 tsp allspice

1 tsp ground cinnamon

4½ pounds lamb shoulder, cubed

1 tbsp butter

6 pearl onions, peeled and halved

12 dried cherries, halved

2 tbsp olive oi

Directions:

Prepare a water bath and place the Sous Vide in it. Set to 141 F.

Combine well the vinegar, red wine, onions, garlic, lemon zest, brown sugar, caraway seeds, cherry jam, corn flour, curry powder, ginger, salt, allspice, and cinnamon.

Place the lamb in a large vacuum-sealable bag. Release air by the water displacement method, seal and submerge the bag in the water bath. Cook for 8 hours. Before 20 minutes to the end, heat the butter in a saucepan and sauté the pearl onions for 8 minutes until softened. Set aside and allow to cool.

Once the timer has stopped, remove the lamb and pat dry with kitchen towel. Reserve the cooking juices and transfer into a saucepan over medium heat and cook for 10 minutes until reduced by half. Fill the skewer with all the kebab ingredients and roll them. Heat the oil in a grill over high heat and cook the kebabs for 45 seconds per side.

Nutrition: Calories 352, Fat 5, Fiber 3, Carbs 7, Protein 5

Bell Pepper & Lamb Curry

Preparation Time: 30 hours 30 minutes

Cooking Time: 25-75 minutes

Servings: 4

Ingredients:

2 tbsp butter

2 bell peppers, chopped

3 garlic cloves, minced

1 tsp turmeric

1 tsp ground cumin

1 tsp paprika

1 tsp grated fresh ginger

½ tsp salt

2 cardamom pods

2 fresh thyme sprigs

2¼ pounds boneless lamb meat, cubed

1 large onion, chopped

3 tomatoes, chopped

1 tsp allspice

2 tbsp Greek yogurt

1 tbsp chopped fresh cilantro

Directions:

Prepare a water bath and place the Sous Vide in it. Set to 179 F. Combine 1 tbsp of butter, bell peppers, 2 garlic cloves, turmeric, cumin, paprika, ginger, salt, cardamom and thyme. Place the lamb in a vacuum-sealable bag with the butter mixture. Release air by the water displacement method, seal and submerge the bag in the water bath. Cook for 30 hours.

Once the timer has stopped, remove the bag and set aside. Heat the butter in a saucepan over high heat. Put the onion and cook for 4 minutes. Add the remaining garlic and cook for 1 minute more. Reduce the heat and add the tomatoes and allspice. Cook for 2 minutes. Pour the yogurt, the lamb and the cooking juices. Cook for 10-15 minutes. Garnish with cilantro.

Nutrition: Calories 352, Fat 5, Fiber 3, Carbs 7, Protein 5

Goat Cheese Lamb Ribs

Preparation Time: 4 hours 10 minutes

Cooking Time: 25-75 minutes

Servings: 2

Ingredients:

Ribs:

2 half racks lamb ribs

2 tbsp vegetable oil

1 clove garlic, minced

2 tbsp rosemary leaves, chopped

1 tbsp fennel pollen

Salt and black pepper to taste

½ tsp cayenne pepper

To Garnish:

8 oz goat cheese, crumbled

2 oz roasted walnuts, chopped

3 tbsp parsley, chopped

Directions:

Make a water bath, place the Sous Vide in it, and set to
134 F. Mix the listed lamb ingredients except for the

lamb. Pat dry the lamb using a napkin and rub the meat with the spice mixture. Place the meat in a vacuum-sealable bag, release air by the water displacement method, seal and submerge the bag in the water bath. Set the timer for 4 hours.

Once the timer has stopped, remove the bag and remove the lamb. Oil and preheat a grill on high heat. Place the lamb on it and sear to become golden brown. Cut the ribs between the bones. Garnish with goat cheese, walnuts and parsley. Serve with a hot sauce dip.

Nutrition: Calories 352, Fat 5, Fiber 3, Carbs 7, Protein 5

Jalapeño Lamb Roast

Preparation Time: 3 hours

Cooking Time: 25-75 minutes

Servings: 6

Ingredients:

1 ½ tbsp canola oil

1 tbsp black mustard seeds

1 tsp cumin seeds

Salt and black pepper to taste

4 lb. butterflied lamb leg

½ cup mint leaves, chopped

½ cup cilantro leaves, chopped

1 shallot, minced

1 clove garlic, minced

2 red jalapenos, minced

1 tbsp red wine vinegar

1 ½ tbsp olive oil

Directions:

Place a skillet over low heat on a stove top. Add ½ tablespoon of olive oil; once it has heated add cumin and mustard seeds and cook for 1 minute. Turn off heat and transfer seeds to a bowl. Add salt and black pepper. Mix. Spread half of the spice mixture inside the lamb leg and roll it. Secure with a butcher's twine at 1- inch intervals.

Season with salt and pepper and massage. Spread half of the spice mixture evenly over inside of lamb leg, then carefully roll it back up. Make a water bath and place Sous Vide in it. Set to 145 F. Place the lamb leg in vacuum-sealable bag, release air by the water displacement method, seal and submerge it in the water bath. Set the timer for 2 hours 45 minutes and cook.

Make the sauce; add to the cumin mustard mixture shallot, cilantro, garlic, red wine vinegar, mint, red chili. Mix and season with salt and pepper. Place aside. Once the timer has stopped, remove and unseal the bag. Remove the lamb and pat dry using a napkin.

Add canola oil to cast iron, preheat over high heat for 10 minutes. Add lamb and sear to brown on both sides. Remove twine and slice lamb. Serve with sauce.

Nutrition: Calories 352, Fat 5, Fiber 3, Carbs 7, Protein 5

Thyme & Sage Grilled Lamb Chops

Preparation Time: 3 hours 20 minutes

Cooking Time: 25-75 minutes

Servings: 6

Ingredients:

6 tbsp butter

4 tbsp dry white wine

4 tbsp chicken broth

4 fresh thyme sprigs

2 garlic cloves, minced

1½ tsp chopped fresh sage

1½ tsp cumin

6 lamb chops

Salt and black pepper to taste

2 tbsp olive oil

Directions:

Prepare a water bath and place the Sous Vide in it. Set to 134 F.

Heat a pot over medium heat and combine butter, white wine, broth, thyme, garlic, cumin and sage. Cook for

5 minutes. Allow to cool. Season the lamb with salt and pepper. Place in three vacuum-sealable bags with the butter mixture. Release air by the water displacement method, seal and submerge the bags in the water bath. Cook for 3 hours.

Once done, remove the lamb and pat dry with kitchen towel. Brush the chops with the olive oil. Heat a skillet over high heat and sear the lamb for 45 seconds per side. Allow to rest for 5 minutes.

Nutrition: Calories 352, Fat 5, Fiber 3, Carbs 7, Protein 5

Lamb Chops With Basil Chimichurri

Preparation Time: 3 hours 40 minutes

Cooking Time: 25-75 minutes

Servings: 4

Ingredients:

Lamb Chops:

3 lamb racks, frenched

3 cloves garlic, crushed

Salt and black pepper to taste

Basil Chimichurri:

1 ½ cups fresh basil, finely chopped

2 banana shallots, diced

3 cloves garlic, minced

1 tsp red pepper flakes

½ cup olive oil

3 tbsp red wine vinegar

Salt and black pepper to taste

Directions:

Prepare a water bath and place the Sous Vide in it. Set to 140 F. Pat dry the racks with a napkin and rub with pepper and salt. Place meat and garlic in a vacuum-sealable bag, release air by water displacement method and seal the bag. Submerge the bag in the water bath. Set the timer for 2 hours and cook.

Make the basil chimichurri: mix all the listed ingredients in a bowl. Cover with cling film and refrigerate for 1 hour 30 minutes. Once the timer has stopped, remove the bag and open it. Remove the lamb and pat dry using a napkin. Sear with a torch to golden brown. Pour the basil chimichurri on the lamb. Serve with a side of steamed greens.

Nutrition: Calories 352, Fat 5, Fiber 3, Carbs 7, Protein 5

Savory Harissa Lamb Kabobs

Preparation Time: 2 hours 30 minutes

Cooking Time: 25-75 minutes

Servings: 10

Ingredients:

3 tbsp olive oil

4 tsp red wine vinegar

2 tbsp chili paste

2 garlic cloves, minced

1½ tsp ground cumin

1½ tsp ground coriander

1 tsp hot paprika

Salt to taste

1½ pounds boneless lamb shoulder, cubed

1 cucumber, peeled and chopped

Zest and juice of ½ lemon

1 cup Greek-style yogurt

Directions:

Prepare a water bath and place the Sous Vide in it. Set
to 134 F. Combine 2 tbsp of olive oil, vinegar, chili,

garlic, cumin, coriander, paprika and salt. Place the lambs and the sauce in a vacuum-sealable bag. Release air by the water displacement method, seal and submerge the bag in the water bath. Cook for 2 hours.

Once the timer has stopped, remove the lamb and pat dry with kitchen towel. Discard the cooking juices. Mix the cucumber, lemon zest and juice, yogurt, and pressed garlic in a small bowl. Set aside. Fill the skewer with the lamb and roll it.

Heat the oil in a skillet over high heat and cook the skewer for 1-2 minutes per side. Top with the lemon-garlic sauce and serve.

Nutrition: Calories 352, Fat 5, Fiber 3, Carbs 7, Protein 5

Duck Leg Confit

Preparation Time: 10-12 hours, Cooking time: 12 hours 10 minutes

Servings: 2

Ingredients:

2 duck legs

1 tbsp dried thyme

2 big bay leaves, crushed

6 tbsp duck fat

Salt and pepper to taste

Cranberry sauce for serving

Directions:

Preheat your Sous Vide machine to 167ºF.

Mix the bay leaves with salt, pepper and thyme, and season the duck legs with the mixture.

Refrigerate overnight.

In the morning, rinse the legs with cold water and carefully put them into the vacuum bag.

Add 4 tbsp duck fat, seal the bag removing the air as much as possible, put it into the water bath and set the cooking time for 12 hours.

Before serving, roast the legs in 2 remaining tbsp of duck fat until crispy.

Serve with cranberry sauce.

Nutrition: Calories 529, Carbohydrates 15 g, Fats 37 g, Protein 34 g,

Lemon Shrimp and Avocado Bowls

Preparation Time: 10 minutes

Cooking Time: 20 minutes

Servings: 4

Ingredients:

1-pound shrimp, peeled and deveined

Juice of ½ lemon

1 avocado, peeled, pitted and cubed

1 cup baby spinach

A pinch of salt and black pepper to the taste

2 tablespoons ghee, melted

Directions:

In s sous vide bag, mix the shrimp with the lemon juice and the other ingredients, toss, seal the bag, put it into your sous vide machine and cook everything at 126 degrees F for 20 minutes.

Divide into bowls and serve for lunch.

Nutrition: Calories 211, Fat 5, Fiber 6, Carbs 12, Protein 6

Mustard Salmon Steaks

Preparation Time: 10 minutes

Cooking Time: 25 minutes

Servings: 4

Ingredients:

4 salmon steaks, bones removed

2 tablespoons mustard

Salt and black pepper to the taste

1 tablespoon lemon juice

1 teaspoon chives, chopped

2 tablespoons olive oil

Directions:

In a bowl, mix the salmon with the mustard and the other ingredients, and toss well.

Transfer the salmon steaks to sous vide bags, seal them, submerge in your sous vide machine and cook at 130 degrees F for 25 minutes.

Divide steaks between plates and serve with a side salad.

Nutrition: Calories 221, Fat 4, Fiber 6, Carbs 12, Protein 5

Balsamic Calamari and Tomatoes

Preparation Time: 10 minutes

Cooking Time: 30 minutes

Servings: 2

Ingredients:

- 1 cup calamari rings
- ½ cup tomato sauce
- 1 cup cherry tomatoes, halved
- 1 teaspoon chili powder
- 4 scallions, chopped
- ½ teaspoon balsamic vinegar
- A pinch of salt and black pepper

Directions:

In a sous vide bag, mix the calamari rings with the tomatoes and the other ingredients, toss, seal the bag, submerge in the water bath and cook at 170 degrees F for 30 minutes.

Divide into bowls and serve for lunch.

Nutrition: Calories 152, Fat 6, Fiber 2, Carbs 6, Protein 5

BBQ Cod Mix

Preparation Time: 10 minutes

Cooking Time: 30 minutes

Servings: 2

Ingredients:

- 1-pound cod fillets, boneless
- 2 tablespoon chives, chopped
- ½ teaspoon coriander, ground
- 1 tablespoon olive oil
- 1 tablespoons BBQ sauce
- 1 tablespoon lime juice
- A pinch of salt and black pepper

Directions:

In a bowl, mix the cod with the BBQ sauce and the other ingredients, toss gently and transfer to a sous vide bag.

Seal the bag, introduce in the preheated water oven and cook at 140 degrees F for 30 minutes.

Divide between plates and serve for lunch.

Nutrition: Calories 200, Fat 6, Fiber 6, Carbs 12, Protein 6

Calamari, Salmon and Shrimp Bowls

Preparation Time: 10 minutes

Cooking Time: 50 minutes

Servings: 4

Ingredients:

- 1 carrot, peeled and sliced
- 1 cup calamari rings
- 1 cup smoked salmon, skinless, boneless and cut into strips
- 1 cup shrimp, peeled and deveined
- 1 celery stalk, chopped
- 1 tablespoon black peppercorns
- 1 garlic clove, minced
- ¼ cup vinegar
- 1 shallot, chopped
- 1 teaspoon mustard
- Juice of 1 lime
- 1 teaspoon smoked paprika
- 1 tablespoon olive oil
- Salt and black pepper to the taste

Directions:

In a sous vide bag, combine the carrot with the calamari and the other ingredients, toss, seal, submerge in the water oven and cook at 185 degrees F for 50 minutes. Divide into bowls and serve.

Nutrition: Calories 215, Fat 4, Fiber 8, Carbs 12, Protein 4

Mustard Salmon Mix

Preparation Time: 10 minutes

Cooking Time: 35 minutes

Servings: 4

Ingredients:

- 1-pound salmon fillets, boneless and roughly cubed
- 2 tablespoons mustard
- 1 cup baby spinach
- 1 cup baby kale
- Salt and black pepper to the taste
- 1 tablespoon homemade mayonnaise
- Juice of 1 lemon
- Zest of 1 lemon, grated
- 2 scallions, chopped
- 2 tablespoons capers, chopped
- 2 tablespoons olive oil

Directions:

In a sous vide bag, combine the salmon with the spinach, mustard and the other ingredients, seal the bag, submerge in the water oven and cook at 170 degrees F for 35 minutes.

Divide into bowls serve.

Nutrition: Calories 201, Fat 3, Fiber 6, Carbs 8, Protein 6

FISH AND SEAFOODS

Standing Rib Roast

Preparation Time: 15 mins

Cooking Time: 24-36 hours

Servings: 4

Ingredients:

1 x 3-rib standing rib roast (6-8 pounds (a.k.a. prime rib roast

1-2 ounces dried morel mushrooms

kosher salt and freshly cracked black pepper, to taste

3 ounces garlic-infused olive oil

Directions:

Attach the sous vide immersion circulator using an adjustable clamp to a Cambro container or pot filled with water and preheat to 130°F.

Into a cooking pouch, add rib roast and mushrooms. Seal pouch tightly after squeezing out the excess air. Place pouch in sous vide bath and set the cooking time for at least 24 and up to 36 hours.

Remove pouch from sous vide bath and carefully open it. Transfer rib roast onto a cutting board, reserve mushroom and cooking liquid into a bowl. With paper towels, pat rib roast completely dry.

Rub rib roast with salt and black pepper evenly.

Heat cast iron pan to medium high heat and place the rib roast in, Fat cap down. Sear for 1-2 minutes per side (or until browned on all sides.

Meanwhile, season reserved mushroom mixture with garlic oil, a little salt, and black pepper.

Transfer rib roast onto a cutting board, bone side down.

Carefully, remove rib bones and cut rib roast into ½-inch-thick slices across the grain.

Serve immediately with mushroom mixture.

Nutrition: Calories 352, Fat 5, Fiber 3, Carbs 7, Protein 5

Best Prime Rib Roast

Preparation Time: 15 mins

Cooking Time: 3 days

Servings: 4

Ingredients:

1 x 10-pound prime rib roast

prime rib spice rub, to taste

dried rosemary, to taste

dried thyme, to taste

onion powder, to taste

garlic powder, to taste

kosher salt and freshly ground black pepper, to taste

Directions:

Attach the sous vide immersion circulator using an adjustable clamp to a Cambro container or pot filled with water and preheat to 135°F.

Carefully, cut individual ribs from the roast.

In a bowl, mix together spice rub, dried herbs, spices, salt and black pepper.

Generously coat roast with spice mixture.

Lightly coat ribs with spice mixture.

Into a cooking pouch, add the roast. In another cooking pouch, place ribs. Seal pouches tightly after squeezing out the excess air. Place pouches in sous vide bath. Each pouch will cook for a different time to allow for maximum tenderness for each cut of meat.

After 5-10 hours, remove roast from sous vide bath and serve. Grass fed or younger, more tender beef will only take 5 hours, while other cuts may take up to 10 hours to become truly tender.

The cuts of ribs can remain in the sous vide bath for up to 72 hours before being removed and served.

Nutrition: Calories 352, Fat 5, Fiber 3, Carbs 7, Protein 5

Korean Short Ribs

Preparation Time: 15 mins

Cooking Time: 4 hours (sous vide then 15 mins

Servings: 4

Ingredients:

For Barbecue Sauce:

1 scallion, finely chopped

6 garlic cloves, crushed

1 tablespoon fresh ginger, grated

1½ cups soy sauce

1½ cups brown sugar

½ cup mirin

½ cup water plus 2 tablespoons water, divided

3 tablespoons chili paste

2 tablespoons rice wine vinegar

1 tablespoon sesame oil

1 teaspoon black pepper, freshly ground

2 tablespoons cornstarch

2 tablespoons water

For Ribs:

4 x 8-ounce boneless beef short ribs

½ teaspoon salt

½ teaspoon black pepper, freshly ground

Directions:

Attach the sous vide immersion circulator using an adjustable clamp to a Cambro container or pot filled with water and preheat to 130°F.

For the barbecue sauce:

in a small bowl, dissolve the cornstarch into 2 tablespoons of water. Keep aside.

In a large pan, mix together remaining sauce ingredients and bring to a boil and cook for 5-7 minutes, stirring occasionally.

Slowly add cornstarch mixture, beating continuously.

Reduce heat to medium and cook for 3-4 minutes.

Remove from heat and keep aside.

For the ribs:

lightly season ribs with salt and black pepper.

Into a cooking pouch, add 1 short rib and 2 tablespoons of barbecue sauce and toss to coat.

Repeat with remaining ribs in separate cooking pouches, and reserve remaining sauce.

Seal pouches tightly after squeezing out the excess air. Place pouches in sous vide bath and set the cooking time for 4 hours.

Remove pouches from sous vide bath and carefully open them. Remove ribs from pouches. With paper towels, pat ribs completely dry.

Heat a cast iron grill pan over high heat, and sear ribs for 10-15 seconds.

Remove ribs from pan and keep aside for 5-10 minutes to rest.

Cut into thin slices and serve immediately with reserved barbecue sauce.

Nutrition: Calories 352, Fat 5, Fiber 3, Carbs 7, Protein 5

Teriyaki Beef Cubes

Preparation Time: 10 minutes

Cooking Time: 60 minutes

Servings: 2

Ingredients:

2 fillet mignon steaks

½ cup teriyaki sauce (extra 6 tablespoons

2 tablespoons soy sauce

2 teaspoons fresh chilis, chopped

1½ tablespoons sesame seeds, toasted

Rice noodles

2 tablespoons sesame oil

1 tablespoon scallion for garnishing, finely chopped

Directions:

Prepare the Sous Vide water bath using your immersion circulator and raise the temperature to 134-degrees Fahrenheit

Slice the steaks into small portions and put them in a zipper bag

Add ½ a cup of teriyaki sauce to the bag. Seal using the immersion method, submerge and cook for 1 hour.

Add the soy sauce and chopped chilis in a small bowl

Add the sesame seeds in another bowl

After 50 minutes of cooking, start cooking the rice noodles according to the package's instructions

Once done, drain the noodles and put them on a servings platter

Take the bag out from the water and remove the beef. Discard the marinade

Take a large skillet and put it over a high heat. Add your sesame oil and allow the oil to heat up.

Add the beef and 6 tablespoons of teriyaki sauce, and cook for 5 seconds

Transfer the cooked beef to your servings platter and garnish with toasted sesame seeds and scallions

Serve with the prepped chili-soy dip

Nutrition: Calories 334, Fat 33, Fiber 3, Carbs 14, Protein 7

POULTRY

Cinnamon Chicken

Preparation Time: 10 minutes

Cooking Time: 1 hour

Servings: 4

Ingredients:

- 2 pounds chicken breasts, skinless, boneless and sliced
- 1 tablespoon cinnamon powder
- 2 tablespoons lemon juice
- ¼ cup chicken stock
- 2 tablespoons avocado oil
- 3 scallions, chopped
- A pinch of salt and black pepper
- 1 teaspoon chili powder
- 2 tablespoons cilantro, chopped

Directions:

In a sous vide bag, mix the chicken with the cinnamon, lemon juice, stock and the other ingredients, toss, seal the bag and cook in the water oven at 170 degrees F for 1 hour.

Divide the mix between plates and serve.

Nutrition: Calories 364, Fat 23.2, Fiber 2.3, Carbs 5.1, Protein 35.4

Turkey Meatballs and Sauce

Preparation Time: 10 minutes

Cooking Time: 55 minutes

Servings: 4

Ingredients:

1-pound turkey breasts, skinless, boneless and ground

2 eggs, whisked

1 red onion, sliced

A pinch of salt and black pepper

1 tablespoon almond flour

2 tablespoons oregano, chopped

1 cup tomato sauce

Directions:

In a bowl, combine the turkey with the onion, eggs, flour salt and pepper, stir and shape medium meatballs out of this mix.

In a sous vide bag, mix the meatballs with the oregano and sauce, seal the bag and cook in the water bath at 170 degrees F for 55 minutes.

Divide the mix between plates and serve.

Nutrition: Calories 300, Fat 15.8, Fiber 2, Carbs 5.2, Protein 33.9

Chicken and Bulgur

Preparation Time: 10 minutes

Cooking Time: 1 hour

Servings: 4

Ingredients:

1-pound chicken breast, skinless, boneless and cubed

1 cup bulgur

1 cup chicken stock

A pinch of salt and black pepper

½ teaspoon coriander, ground

1 teaspoon turmeric powder

1 tablespoon chives, chopped

Directions:

In a sous vide bag, mix the chicken with the bulgur, stock and the other ingredients, seal the bag and cook in the water bath at 170 degrees F for 1 hour.

Divide the mix between plates and serve.

Nutrition: Calories 360, Fat 22.1, Fiber 1.4, Carbs 4.3, Protein 34.5

Turkey and Tomatoes

Preparation Time: 10 minutes

Cooking Time: 1 hour

Servings: 4

Ingredients:

2 pounds turkey breasts, skinless, boneless and cubed

½ pound cherry tomatoes, halved

Juice of 1 lime

1 tablespoon balsamic vinegar

1 tablespoon avocado oil

½ teaspoon smoked paprika

A pinch of salt and black pepper

1 tablespoon cilantro, chopped

Directions:

In a sous vide bag, mix the turkey with the tomatoes, lime juice and the other ingredients, seal the bag and cook in the water bath at 180 degrees F for 1 hour. Divide between plates and serve.

Nutrition: Calories 362, Fat 16.1, Fiber 4.4, Carbs 5.4, Protein 36.4

Turkey with Spinach and Kale

Preparation Time: 10 minutes

Cooking Time: 1 hour

Servings: 4

Ingredients:

2 pounds turkey breasts, skinless, boneless and cubed

2 tablespoons olive oil

1 cup baby spinach

1 cup baby kale

Juice of 1 lime

¼ cup white wine

4 garlic cloves, minced

1 tablespoon lime zest, grated

A pinch of salt and black pepper

1 tablespoon parsley, chopped

Directions:

In a sous vide bag, mix the turkey with the oil, spinach and the other ingredients, seal the bag, cook in the water bath at 175 degrees F for 1 hour, divide everything between plates and serve.

Nutrition: Calories 243, Fat 9, Fiber 1.6, Carbs 5.4,

Protein 34.1

Turkey and Spring Onions

Preparation Time: 10 minutes

Cooking Time: 50 minutes

Servings: 4

Ingredients:

2 pounds turkey breast, skinless, boneless and cubed

1 cup spring onions, chopped

¼ cup white wine

½ teaspoon sweet paprika

½ teaspoon chili powder

2 tablespoons avocado oil

1 tablespoon parsley, chopped

A pinch of salt and black pepper

Directions:

In a large sous vide bag, mix the turkey with the spring onions, wine and the other ingredients, seal the bag, submerge in the water bath, cook at 175 degrees F for 50 minutes, divide the mix between plates and serve.

Nutrition: Calories 222, Fat 6.7, Fiber 1.6, Carbs 4.8,

Protein 34.4

Chicken and Lime Red Cabbage

Preparation Time: 10 minutes

Cooking Time: 1 hour

Servings: 4

Ingredients:

1-pound chicken breasts, skinless, boneless and cubed

1 cup red cabbage, shredded

Juice of 1 lime

Zest of 1 lime, grated

2 tablespoons olive oil

2 tablespoons balsamic vinegar

A pinch of salt and black pepper

1 tablespoon chives, chopped

1 tablespoon rosemary, chopped

Directions:

In a large sous vide bag, mix the chicken with the cabbage, lime juice and the other ingredients, seal the bag, submerge in the water bath, cook at 180 degrees F for 1 hour, divide between plates and serve.

Nutrition: Calories 264, Fat 13.2, Fiber 0.7, Carbs 1.9, Protein 33.2

SNACKS & DESSERTS

Pecan Plums Bowls

Preparation time: 10 minutes

Cooking time: 35 minutes

Servings: 4

Ingredients:

½ teaspoon vanilla extract

Juice of 1 lime

2 tablespoons sugar

½ teaspoon cinnamon powder

1 pound plums, stoned and halved

½ cups pecans, chopped

1 cup heavy cream

Directions:

In a sous vide bag, mix the plums with the pecans, cream and the other ingredients, toss, seal the bag, submerge in the preheated water oven and cook at 183 degrees F for 35 minutes.

Divide into bowls and serve.

Nutrition: calories 152 fat 2 fiber 2 carbs 8 protein 7

Rhubarb Jam and Blackberry

Preparation time: 10 minutes

Cooking time: 50 minutes

Servings: 4

Ingredients:

1 pound blackberries

2 cups rhubarb, chopped

2 cups water

Juice of 1 lime

1 cup sugar

Directions:

In a sous vide bag, mix the berries with the rhubarb and the other ingredients, whisk, seal the bag, submerge it in the preheated water oven and cook at 185 degrees F for 1 hour.

Divide into cups and serve cold.

Nutrition: calories 100 fat 2 fiber 3 carbs 8 protein 3

Black Currant Marmalade

Preparation time: 2 hours

Cooking time: 1 hour

Servings: 8

Ingredients:

Juice of 1 lemon

Zest of 1 lemon, grated

2 tablespoon water

½ pound blueberries

4 ounces black currant

2 cups sugar

Directions:

In a sous vide bag, mix the berries with the currant and the other ingredients, whisk, seal the bag, submerge it in the preheated water oven and cook at 180 degrees F for 1 hour.

Divide into bowls and keep in the fridge for 2 hours before serving.

Nutrition: calories 100 fat 2 fiber 3 carbs 7 protein 3

Lime Jam

Preparation time: 10 minutes

Cooking time: 45 minutes

Servings: 8

Ingredients:

   2 tablespoons lime zest, grated

   2 tablespoons lime juice

   1 cup sugar

   1 cup water

   1 tablespoon ginger, grated

Directions:

In a sous vide bag, mix the lime juice with the sugar and the other ingredients, seal the bag, submerge it in the preheated water oven and cook at 160 degrees F for 45 minutes.

Divide into bowls and serve cold.

Nutrition: calories 162 fat 2 fiber 3 carbs 8 protein 4

Creamy Pears

Preparation time: 10 minutes

Cooking time: 50 minutes

Servings: 6

Ingredients:

1 pound, cored and cut into quarters

1 cup heavy cream

¼ cup apple juice

1 teaspoon cinnamon powder

½ teaspoon nutmeg, ground

Directions:

In a sous vide bag, mix the pears with the cream and the other ingredients, seal the bag, submerge it in the preheated water oven and cook at 180 degrees F for 50 minutes.

Divide into bowls and serve cold.

Nutrition: calories 100 fat 2 fiber 2 carbs 6 protein 4

Peaches Bowls

Preparation time: 10 minutes

Cooking time: 30 minutes

Servings: 6

Ingredients:

½ teaspoon cinnamon powder

1 teaspoon vanilla extract

1 cup heavy cream

6 peaches, cored and cut into quarters

3 tablespoons sugar

Directions:

In a sous vide bag, mix the peaches with the sugar and the other ingredients, seal the bag, submerge it in the preheated water bath and cook at 183 degrees F for 30 minutes.

Divide into bowls and serve.

Nutrition: calories 125 fat 3 fiber 5 carbs 6 protein 4